Feeding with Love
and Good Sense:
18 Months through 6 Years

**Feeding with Love and Good Sense:
18 Months through 6 Years**

Copyright © 2020 by Ellyn Satter

kelcy press

All rights reserved. No part of this book may be reproduced or transmitted in any form or by any means, electronic or mechanical, including photocopying and recording or by any information storage and retrieval, without permission in writing from Ellyn Satter.

ISBN 978-0-9908975-2-1

Developmental editor, Nancy Pekar

Part of the five-part series

Feeding with Love and Good Sense: The First Two Years
Feeding with Love and Good Sense: 18 months through 6 years
Feeding with Love and Good Sense: 6 to 13 years
Feeding with Love and Good Sense: 12 to 18 years
Feeding Yourself *with Love and Good Sense*

Show this booklet to your health care provider!

Encourage purchasing in bulk for office or classroom
Discounts up to 50%

Distributed by
Ellyn Satter Institute
www.EllynSatterInstitute.org
esi@EllynSatterInstitute.org

Feeding with Love and Good Sense:

18 Months through 6 Years

Ellyn Satter
Nutritionist and Family Therapist

Table of Contents

1. **Raise a healthy child who is a joy to feed** 1
   You can have enjoyable, harmonious meals. Your child can be healthy, feel good about eating, and behave well around food.

2. **Follow the division of responsibility** 3
   To raise a healthy child who eats and grows well, do your jobs with feeding and parenting, then trust your child to do her jobs with eating, moving, and growing.

3. **Understand your child's development** 9
   Consider the toddler, the preschooler, and the school-age child. Being able to recognize stages in development and understand temperament lets you trust and enjoy your child and parent in the best way.

4. ***How* to feed your child** 13
   Have family-friendly meals (page 15) and sit-down snacks (page 26). The toddler's eating is quirky (page 16), the preschooler's eating is surprising (page 18), and the school-age child's eating skills start to show (page 20). Look forward to greater mealtime tranquility as your child gets older.

5. ***What* to feed your family** 25
   You are now feeding a *family* and including your child in *family meals*. You are no longer just feeding your child.

6. **Solve feeding problems** 31
   Consider the picky eater, the child who doesn't eat meals and then begs for food, the large child, the small child, the child who doesn't eat much, the child who doesn't eat vegetables or drink milk, or the child with special needs.

7. **What you have learned** 39
   Feeding is parenting in all ways. You have to do your jobs, but then you have to let go. Throughout the growing-up years, maintain a division of responsibility in feeding.

Dedication: This booklet is dedicated to you, the parent, and all the caring adults who are helping feed your child with love and good sense.

A message from Ellyn Satter

If all has gone well for you up until now, you have successfully navigated a lot of pitfalls with respect to feeding your child:

- Your child happily ate solid food. Or he didn't. But you were able to stay relaxed. You learned that some children don't get interested in solids until they can finger-feed themselves.
- One day he refused to let you feed him and grabbed for the spoon. Through careful observation and deduction or sheer luck, you correctly figured out that he wanted to feed himself. Resisting the entirely natural response to play "here comes the airplane," you let him.
- She enthusiastically ate with her fingers almost everything that was offered. She loved joining in with family meals.
- Suddenly, he got picky. He ate very little, was skeptical of food that he had eaten many times before, and reacted to the mildest suggestion about food as if you were Attila the Hun (with apologies to all Huns everywhere). Being by now a seasoned observer, you resisted the impulse to make special food or try to get him to eat, and correctly interpreted this behavior as being natural for a toddler.
- Again suddenly, you sail into quiet waters. After months of skirmishing around food and everything else, your child becomes a preschooler and then a school-age child. She is more willing to try new food and it is relaxing to have her at family meals. There are pitfalls to come, but you can handle them!

On the other hand, you, like a lot of other parents, may have fallen into the pitfalls rather than steering around them. You are left with food hassles or with a child who eats only a *short* list of foods. Family meals may be so unpleasant that you consider giving up on them.

It is not too late! Your child is still very young. If you change your ways with feeding and *keep* them changed, your child will become a good eater, and you will enjoy feeding. This booklet tells you how.

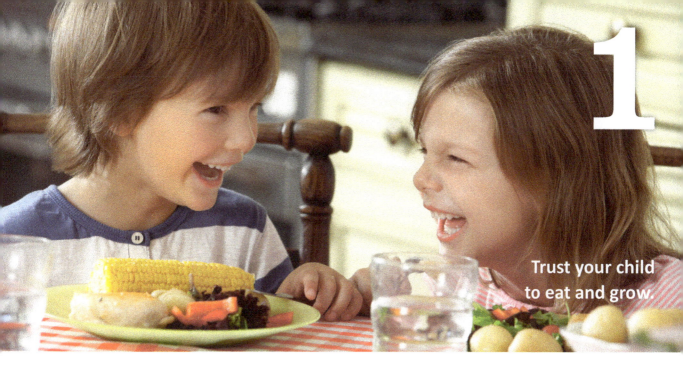

Trust your child to eat and grow.

1. Raise a healthy child who is a joy to feed

A good eater is a *competent* eater. Focus on *how* you feed and *how* your child behaves at mealtime, not on *what* your child eats. When you maintain the quality of your feeding relationship rather than worrying about your child's food consumption, you will trust him to eat and grow well. Sooner or later, he will learn to eat almost everything you eat. In the meantime, understand and expect normal child eating behavior. It is normal for your child to be a picky eater, to eat only one or two foods from any meal, to eat a food one time and ignore it another, to eat a lot one time and not much another, and to not eat vegetables.

You can make up for past feeding mistakes

If your child is *not* a competent eater, do not despair. Follow the guidelines in this booklet and all will be well. He is still very young, and when you change your ways with feeding and *keep* them changed, he will change his ways with eating.

Your child is a competent eater when . . .

- **He feels good about eating.** He enjoys food and joins in happily with family meals and snacks.

- **He enjoys meals and behaves nicely at mealtime.** He feels good about being included in family meals and does his part to make mealtime pleasant. He does not make a fuss.

- **He picks and chooses from food you eat with only minor chewing/swallowing/seasoning changes.** He is okay with being offered food he has never seen before. He ignores food he does not want and also "sneaks up" on new food and learns to eat it. Eventually he will learn to eat almost everything you do.

- **He eats as much or as little as he needs.** Only he knows how much that is. Trusting him to eat as much he needs lets him grow consistently and develop the body that nature intended for him.

Do your jobs with feeding and let your child do her jobs with eating

- Follow the division of responsibility (next page). You do the *what, when* and *where* of *feeding* and trust your child to do the *how much* and *whether* of *eating*.
- Trust your child to grow in the way that is right for her.
- *Understand your child's development* (page 9). Feed—and parent—in the way that is right for each stage.
- *Solve feeding problems* (page 31) by applying what you have learned in this booklet.

Your child will be healthy and grow well

When you follow the division of responsibility and your child feels good about eating, she will eat as much as she needs, grow in the way that is right for her, and, over time, learn to eat a variety of food. You may feel, however, that it is your job to "get in" nutritious food or get your child to eat a certain amount and grow in a certain way. By comparison, following the division of responsibility may seem like doing nothing at all. In reality, keeping up the day-in-and-day-out of pleasant and rewarding *family meals* (page 15) and *sit-down snacks* (page 26) is doing a tremendous amount. Parents say that following the division of responsibility *works* (page 6).

The division of responsibility applies to *your* special child

Every child is unusual in some way. The division of responsibility applies to all children and applies to children of all ages, birth through adolescence. The problem is that some children's characteristics and behaviors make it seem that they can't be trusted to do their part with eating. They can. With some children more than others, sticking to the division of responsibility demands steady nerves and a leap of faith. Here is help:

- The child who won't eat family meals (page 32).
- The "too-small" child who seemingly doesn't eat enough (page 34).
- The "too-big child" who seemingly eats too much (page 33).
- The picky eater (page 31).
- The child who doesn't eat vegetables (page 35) or drink milk (page 36).
- The child with special needs (page 37).

My toddler is a joy to feed

As a dietitian, I have studied Ellyn Satter's books and watched the *Feeding with Love and Good Sense Videos* as well so that I can counsel parents. But only since I have had a child of my own have I fully realized the importance of the division of responsibility. My husband and I look forward to mealtime with our busy toddler. My son runs eagerly to the table when we call him and we all enjoy eating together. It is so much fun to watch him eat! We let him eat whatever he wants in the meal and do not coax him to eat anything else. Our friends are amazed at how well he eats in general and how pleasant he is at the table. I am so thankful for the joy and relaxation we are able to experience at our family meals. I know it is due to the fact that we are following Ellyn Satter's philosophy—we do our jobs and we let him do his.

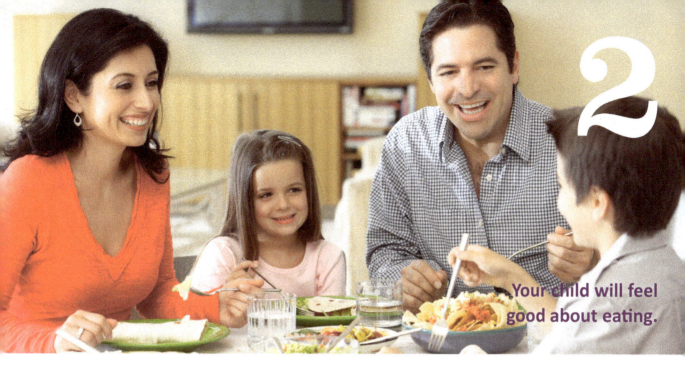

Your child will feel good about eating.

2. Follow the division of responsibility

The best way to feed your child—no matter her age—is to follow the *division of responsibility*. As a parent, you provide *structure, support,* and *opportunities to learn*. Your child chooses *how much* and *whether to* eat from what you provide. The division of responsibility in feeding encourages you to take leadership with feeding and give your child autonomy with eating.

THE DIVISION OF RESPONSIBILITY
toddlers through adolescents

- You are responsible for **what, when,** and **where** to feed your child.
- Your child is responsible for **how much** and **whether** to eat of the foods you put before her.

Do your feeding jobs:

- Choose and serve the food. Provide regular meals and snacks.
- Make eating times pleasant.
- Show your child how to behave at meals.
- Maintain structure. Offer your child water between regular meal- and snack-times but not other drinks or food.
- Let your child grow in her way.

Trust your child to do her eating jobs:

- She will eat.
- She will eat the amount she needs.
- She will learn to eat the food you eat.
- She will learn to behave well at family meals.
- She will grow up to have the body that is right for her.

Trust your child to grow in the best way

Your child has a natural way of growing that is right for her. Her natural growth is in balance with her eating and moving. Maintain the division of responsibility in feeding and in activity *(next page)*. Trust her to do her part with eating, moving, and growing.

Your child's body shape and size are mostly inherited. The amounts she needs to eat are also inherited, and support her growing and moving in her own unique way. Her height and weight are normal for her as long as she grows consistently, even if her growth plots at the extreme upper or lower ends of the growth charts. Don't let anyone make an issue of your child's size, shape or weight, and beware of hidden messages. Children who are encouraged to eat or move in a certain way to be "healthy" get the idea that there is something wrong with their body. They feel flawed in every way: not smart, not physically capable, and not worthy.

You won't know how your child's body will turn out until she is toward the end of her teen years and even beyond. Trying to control or change it will likely create the very outcome you are trying to avoid! As long as you keep your nerve and maintain the division of responsibility with feeding and with activity, her growth may surprise you. The fat child is likely to slim down. The small, ill, or growth-delayed child is likely to continue to do catch-up growth well into her teen years and has a good chance of being bigger than you may expect.

If your child's weight or height *abruptly* shifts up or down on her growth chart, it can mean there is a problem. Consult a health professional who understands the feeding relationship to rule out feeding, health, or parenting problems.

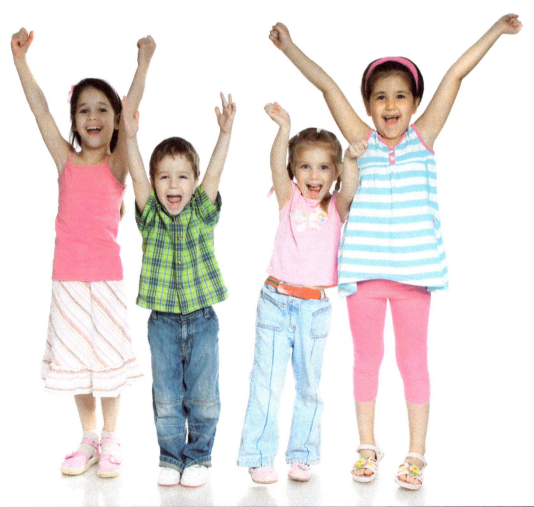

Follow the division of responsibility in activity

As with feeding, do your jobs and let your children do theirs. You don't have to *make* children be active. They are born loving their bodies. They are curious about their physical capabilities and inclined to be active in a way that is right for them. Each child is naturally more or less skilled, graceful, energetic, or aggressive. Good parenting with activity preserves those qualities and lets a child be all she can be.

The division of responsibility in activity

- You are responsible for *structure, safety,* and *opportunities*.
- Your child is responsible for *how, how much,* and *whether* she moves.

Do your jobs

- Develop your tolerance for commotion—and your judgment about how much is too much.
- Provide safe places for activity your child enjoys.
- Find fun and rewarding family activities.
- Set limits on TV and other media but not on reading, writing, artwork, or other quiet activities.
- Don't let your child have a TV set or streaming device in her room.
- Don't try to entertain your child—let her deal with her own boredom.

Trust your child to do her jobs

- Your child will be active.
- She will be active in a way that is right for her.
- Her physical capabilities will grow and develop.
- She will experiment and find activities that she enjoys and that are in concert with her capabilities.

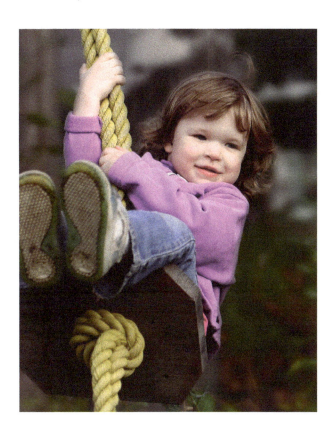

The division of responsibility works

I fought about vegetables with my preschooler

Our four-year-old, Kevin, ate very few foods and he especially didn't eat vegetables! So we tried to get him to eat vegetables and not so many carbohydrates and to eat more if we thought he hadn't eaten enough and to stop eating when we thought he was eating too much. Every meal was such a hassle that we were about to give up on meals! But since we started going by the division of responsibility in feeding we have stress-free meals—and snacks, of course. Kevin is so much happier, and so are we.

Grady grew slowly

Grady had always been long and lean, but at his three-year-old checkup his weight had dropped below his usual third percentile and my pediatrician recommended appetite-stimulating medication. That didn't sound right to me. I asked him to give me 3 months and a referral to a dietitian. She helped me realize I had been putting pressure on Grady to eat and generally not making eating enjoyable for him, and recommended I read *Secrets of Feeding a Healthy Family*. What a relief to realize I only had to be responsible for providing healthy, balanced meals and snacks, and I could let Grady be responsible for eating. Grady gained weight, I shed my stress over food, and now we all eat better.

I had to let Henry get hungry

I thought I was following the division of responsibility in feeding, but between meals I let my two-year-old, Henry, eat whenever he wanted to. The food was healthy—I hauled little bags of crackers and juice boxes along so he could eat whenever he felt a hunger pang. Then I learned about the *sit-down snack*! Henry was no longer a baby who had to be fed on demand. He could last 2 or 3 hours before he had to eat again. At first, he put up a fuss when I stopped giving him food handouts, but before long he got used to having his snacks at certain times. Getting a little hungry before meals makes him eat better. And I no longer have cracker crumbs and juice smears all over the house and car!

My son has autism

My seven-year-old son, Gabe, was diagnosed with high-functioning autism when he was three. He has always been a super-cautious eater, first with breastfeeding, then semi-solid foods, and now table food. We are told that he has Sensory Processing Disorder, meaning that he is really sensitive to tastes and textures, and we were told, "stop coddling him and make him eat." I am not proud of all our begging, pleading, pressuring, forcing, cajoling, and rewarding! But Ellyn Satter reassured me that we could follow the division of responsibility, even with Gabe. So we did. I always put something on the table he usually ate—applesauce, bread and butter—something that went along with the meal and didn't involve making him his own meal. At first he had tantrums when we wouldn't make what he wanted, but compared with before, this was *easy*! Gabe is still a "picky" eater, but he does his part to make mealtime pleasant by settling happily for what I put on the table, even if he isn't enthusiastic about it.

Structure is essential

Your child will eat and grow well if you maintain structure. To provide structure for your child, you have to provide structure for yourself. Have a schedule for sit-down meals and sit-down snacks. Stick to it.

Structure supports both you and your child

Structure lets both you and your child know you will be fed. Structure helps you each to eat what and how much your body needs. Don't wait until hunger drives you to figure out what to eat. You will grab for the first food at hand, and whether you know it or not, you will scare yourself into overeating—and you will scare your child, as well.

Meals do not have to be a chore or a bore

- *Have family-friendly meals* (page 15). Provide food you enjoy.
- *Have sit-down snacks* (page 26) **between meals.** A planned snack between meals lets you and your child arrive at mealtime hungry and ready to eat. Drinking (except for water) and munching between times spoils meals.
- **Avoid feeding struggles.** They will spoil your meals. Follow the division of responsibility.
- **Make family meals pleasant.** Your child wants to be at family meals because you are there.
- **Expect your child to contribute.** Joining in with family meals is a privilege that your child earns by behaving nicely.

Be considerate without catering

- **Remember whose meal it is.** You know more about food than your child does. Your child is growing up to learn to eat the food *you* eat and to join in with *your* meals.
- **Make only one meal, but include easy-to-eat foods.** Include one or two foods that your child—and other eaters—generally eat and can fill up on, such as bread or fruit. Don't worry if your child eats it and only it meal after meal, day after day. Eventually he will eat something different.
- **Include fat.** Include fat when you cook, and make it available at mealtime to make food taste good. Fat with food also keeps everyone from getting hungry right away. Your toddler may eat butter as if it were cheese. That's okay. He needs the calories.
- **Trust your child to eat.** He wants to eat, he wants to learn to eat the food you eat, and he will tire of even his favorite food and eat something different. Sooner or later (maybe later rather than sooner) he will eat a variety.
- **Don't take it personally.** Food is love. But your family's *not* eating the food you prepare isn't the same as not accepting your love. Other family members love you back and eat what they enjoy.

Drinking and eating on the go

Keep your feeding goal in mind: Helping your child to *be a competent eater* (page 1), *not* getting-food-into-your-child-right-now. It doesn't matter if the food or drink is nutritious, created especially for children, or even *organic*. Letting your child slurp and munch on the go will keep him from being a competent eater, and his nutrition will suffer. Just like other children, your child is likely to *love* eating and drinking wherever, whenever. But if you let him, expect this: He will have trouble knowing how much he needs to eat and may eat too little and grow too slowly or eat too much and grow too fast. He will behave poorly at family meals because he isn't hungry and can't be bothered. He won't learn to eat the food you eat because *his* special food, delivered in *his* special way, is more to his liking.

Family meals are about *family*

If considering family meals puts you on a guilt trip and makes you feel overwhelmed, skip ahead to *Have family-friendly meals* (page 15). Especially read the section, "prepare food you enjoy." Here is the bottom line: Family meals are first and foremost about *family*. They are not about food virtue: about providing only fresh-cooked food that earns a gold star from the food police.

- Meals give a time and place to provide your child with food and reassure her she will be fed. You can pay attention and enjoy food when it is time to eat, then forget about it between times.
- Meals let you conduct the business of the family, keep up with what is going on with everybody, help each other out, and tell family stories.
- Meals teach your child how to behave at mealtime. That lets you enjoy her, and lets her be comfortable when she eats with other people.
- Both you and your child do better when you have family meals. You learn to enjoy a variety of food. Going to the meal hungry and eating until you get enough supports eating the amount you need and weighing what is right for you.
- Now is the time to get family meals in place! Children and teens who have regular family meals feel better about themselves, get along better with other people, and do better in school. Teens who have family meals are less likely to abuse drugs and have sex.

What is a family?

You are a family when you take care of yourself. Whether your family numbers one or ten, whether you are related or a group of people living together, have family meals.

Sit-down snacks solve feeding problems

Planned, *sit-down snacks* (page 26) are the ace in the hole of the beleaguered parent. When you know a sit-down snack is coming in a couple of hours, you can say, "that's it for now, snack time is coming soon." You can say to your school-aged child, "snack time is now. Sit down and eat now, or you have to wait for dinner." The planned snack solves these feeding problems:

- Your child leaves the meal having eaten little or nothing. He is back 5 minutes later begging for food.
- Your child has eaten well at the meal, but happens to think, "cookie," and starts begging.
- Your child did not eat much and seems okay with that, but *you* worry that he will not make it until the next meal.
- Your child comes home famished, is too busy to take time to eat, and wants to munch along with other activities.
- Your child eats constantly until dinner, in front of the TV or while doing homework.

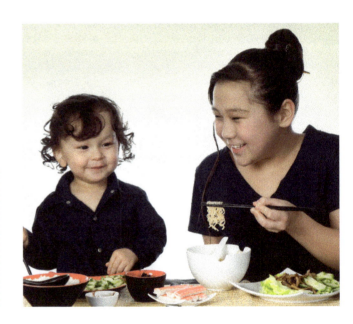

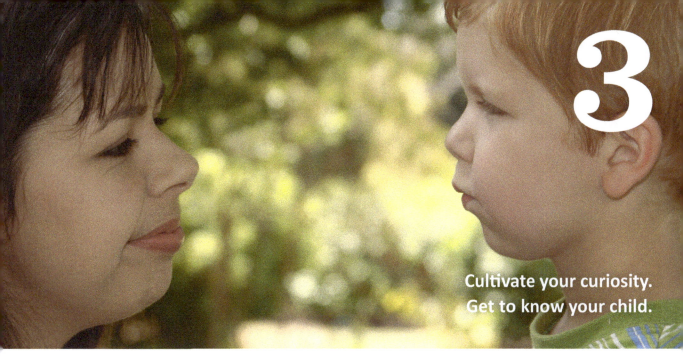

Cultivate your curiosity. Get to know your child.

3. Understand your child's development

Being able to recognize and understand your child's stages in development lets you trust and enjoy him and parent in the best way. From 18 months through 6 years, he moves through being a toddler and then a preschooler and becomes an early school-age child. To identify his developmental stage, go by what he *does*, not by his age.

Toddler: 18 months to 3 years

If you are confused about the concept of control—what is yours to control and what is your child's—check in with a toddler. *You* may be vague about the line between your feeding and his eating, but he is *not*. He knows when you are imposing your will on him and puts up a fuss. That is all part of his working on *separation-individuation:* On both being part of your family *and* being his own little person.

Follow the division of responsibility in feeding
Your toddler needs structure in all things, including feeding. Don't drop everything to feed him, as you did when he was a baby. Instead, have him join in with *family meals* (page 15) and provide *sit-down snacks* (page 26) between times. He is learning to wait a bit to eat—and get a bit hungry. Giving him sit-down snacks keeps him from having to wait *too* long or get *too* hungry. The toddler grows more slowly than before, needs fewer calories, and therefore eats less. Hang in there! He will eat what the rest of the family eats, but it has to be *his* idea.

- **Maintain the structure of meals and snacks.** Do not try to get him to eat.
- **Let him ignore the vegetables.** But still include them and enjoy them yourself.
- **Do not give him food handouts.** Ignore his tantrums.
- **Let him eat at a snack time that *you* determine.** Occasionally let him eat as many cookies as he wants.

Managing feeding skirmishes

Toddlers—and older children who act like toddlers—behave in ways that tempt you to do *their* jobs with feeding.

"I'm not hungry." Oscar says "I'm not hungry" when his parents call him to dinner. At first, his parents say, "Oh dear, you *must* be hungry." Then they wise up: his being hungry is *his* business. Having a family meal is *their* business. So, they give him a five-minute warning. Then they say, "You don't have to eat, but come and keep us company while we eat." Sometimes Oscar eats happily for a while and then wants down. Sometimes he doesn't eat at all and wants down after a minute or two. At first, his parents keep him at the table in hopes that he will eat more. But he doesn't, and he makes such a commotion that they realize they have to let him down when he wants down.

"Now I'm hungry." Oscar, having not eaten his meal, is back begging to sit on his daddy's lap and eat off his daddy's plate. When his daddy lets him, Oscar creates a commotion. So, his daddy says, "No, you have had your meal. That's it until snack time." Oscar tries his mother. She tells him the same thing. Oscar has a tantrum. His parents ignore him.

"Let's play." Oscar, having more-or-less eaten his meal and been allowed to get down from the table, is back looking for attention while his parents try to enjoy their meal. They tell him to play, but he continues to pester. At the next meal, they wash Oscar up, clear away his dishes, let him down, put some toys not too far from the table, and spend a minute or two helping him get started playing. Then they go back to eating. They look at him from time to time while he plays and say a word or two. But they don't let him spoil their meal.

Preschooler: 3 years to 5 years

Whew! If all has gone well during the toddler stage, your preschooler is easy to be around. She works on *initiative, impulse regulation,* and *internalization of limits.* She wants to try things out (including eating new food), to learn and do, to understand, to do what you ask, and to please you! She can keep out of trouble, be on her own for short times, and remember your instructions. But she cannot *eat* on her own. She needs you to maintain the division of responsibility in feeding and to eat with her, not just feed her. Compared with when she was a toddler, the preschooler is less skeptical about new food, more willing to try it, and pushes herself more to learn to eat it. But in some ways, that makes feeding harder. You can get her to eat more, less, or different food than she wants. But if you do, it will make her feel ashamed of eating what she doesn't want. If she is not so compliant, she will find pleasing you to be just too difficult, will resist your pressure on her to eat, and feeding will become a battleground. But she loves you as much as ever, and even if she acts angry and defiant, she will feel ashamed of going against your wishes. (See Avoid Pressure on page 23.)

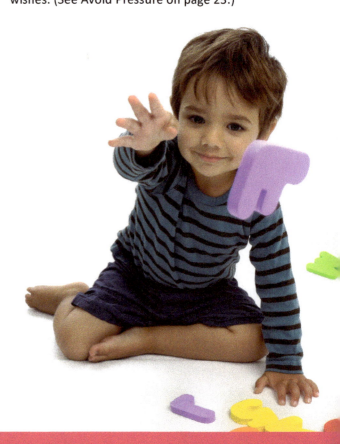

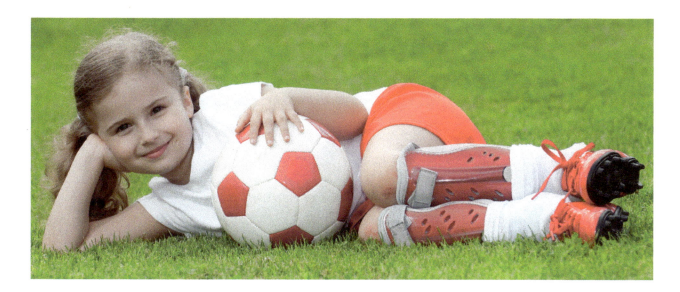

Early school-age child: 5 years through 6 years (and beyond)

Throughout the school-age years, your child works on *industry*. He learns and practices grown-up skills and develops a view of himself as being capable. Because he is so similar to an older and more competent preschooler, he is easy to be around. But his competence can fool you into thinking you are not as important as before. Not so. As long as you back him up, he is positive and curious and wants to learn and do. He attacks a task for the pure joy of being on the move and trying out what the world has to offer. His energy lets him breeze right by setbacks and keep on working at whatever task he sets for himself. If all has gone well earlier on with feeding, the school-age child is secure and comfortable with the division of responsibility. He accepts the meal- and snack-time structure and eats an increasing number of foods. Now as before, and throughout his growing-up years, he knows how much he needs to eat—provided you haven't interfered by getting controlling with feeding. You can pressure your school-age child into eating certain foods, but that will make it a chore for him and take away all his enjoyment. You can also get him to eat certain amounts, but that will take away his knowing how much he needs to eat and interfere with his growing in the way that is right for him.

The cautious, slow-to-warm-up child

How do you deal with a child who is slow to eat or even to try anything new? Do your jobs, and let him take his time. It can take *years*, but if you refrain from getting pushy about his eating, sooner or later he will eat most everything you eat.

- Let your child pick and choose from what you provide for the meal. He might eat only one or two foods.
- Don't force your child to eat—or even to taste—one food before he can have another.
- Don't offer substitutes.
- When you introduce new foods, also offer something familiar that your child eats and can fill up on.
- Serve bread with every meal, and let your child eat as much of it as he wants, even if he doesn't eat anything else.
- Don't give choices on the main dish. Always including peanut butter, cheese, or cereal with the meal tells your child, "I do not expect you to learn to eat what we eat."

Feeding as Parenting

Your child loves you and wants to grow up to be just like you. He wants to learn to eat the food you eat. He will do best when you give him both love and limits—you do your jobs with feeding and let him do his jobs with eating.

What your child wants and needs:	What to do as a parent:
He wants to do well with eating.	Plan meals with both familiar and unfamiliar food. Let him eat or not eat from what you offer.
He needs pleasant mealtimes.	Talk about something else besides food. Help him learn to make conversation. Don't scold.
He needs to feel independent.	Help him get served, then don't interfere. Don't wipe, tidy, arrange, encourage, remind, suggest, or insist.
He wants to eat the same way you do.	Provide him with the same place setting you use—child-sized if you can. Let him learn by watching how you manage your silverware and napkin. Don't pester him—he is doing his best.
He wants to do it himself.	Let him serve himself. Teach him to dish up a little at a time, put the serving spoon back in the bowl, and pass the bowl to the next person. Keep extra spoons handy—learning takes a while!
He needs to know you approve.	Recognize when he does well. But don't make a big deal about it or he will think, "I must be stupid."
He will test the rules.	His behavior is negative if it interferes with your having a pleasant meal. Matter-of-factly tell him to stop. Excuse him from the meal if he persists.

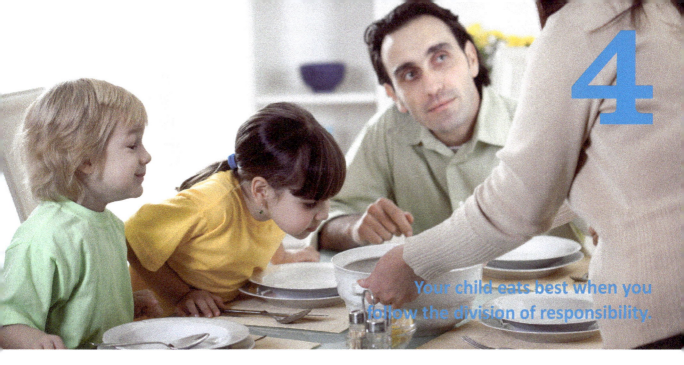

Your child eats best when you follow the division of responsibility.

4. How to feed your child

Look forward to greater mealtime tranquility as your child gets older, but prepare for surprises! How to feed is the essentially the same for the toddler, the preschooler, and the school-age child. What changes is the mess, the commotion, the waste, and your child's voluntarily saying "please," and "may I be excused" after 1001 reminders. At every stage and age, your child will eat best when you maintain a division of responsibility in feeding. You determine the *what, when,* and *where* of *feeding*. Your child determines the *how much* and *whether* of *eating*—from what you provide.

Maintain structure

- **Have *family-friendly meals*** (page 15) and ***sit-down snacks*** (page 26).
  Don't make food available all the time. Don't let her eat or drink on the run. Let her drink water in between times.

- **Have meals and snacks be your idea.**
  Don't wait for her to say "I am hungry" before you offer meals and snacks. Offer the regular sit-down snack even if she forgets about it.

- **Keep control of the menu.**
  Don't ask, "what would you like?" She does not know until it is in front of her, and maybe not even then!

The food

- **Give about a tablespoon per year of age.**
  Don't give her a lot or not enough. Let her have more when she wants it. Don't make her eat one food before she can have another.

- **As soon as she is ready, let her serve herself. Don't fuss about spills.**
  Teach her to take small helpings and ask for more, but don't try to control her portion size. Even when she takes small helpings, don't make her eat what she takes.

- **Keep making food you enjoy—sooner or later she will learn to eat most foods.**
  Don't cook for her—cook for yourself. Don't ask her what she wants you to make—that is *your* job. Don't try in *any way* to make her eat—eating is *her* job.

During the meal

- **Eat with your child. Enjoy your own meal or snack.**
  Don't go off and leave her while she eats.

- **Let her eat her way—fast or slowly, fingers or utensils.**
  Let her eat as fast or slowly as is right for her. Give her silverware and a napkin, but don't insist she use them.

- **Let her eat a lot or a little. Don't try to make her eat more or less.**
  Don't try to get her to taste everything or to take a few more bites. Don't make her stop eating before she is full.

- **Be good company. Be easy-going. Talk about something besides the food and eating.**
  Don't ignore her, but don't make her the center of attention either. Don't read. Turn off all the electronic devices. *All* of them.

- **Teach her to behave so you can have a nice meal. Excuse her when she is done.**
  Don't put up with negative behavior or make her stay at the meal in hopes she will eat.

Understand gagging and choking

Gagging is not a problem. A child gags to push food out when it slips to the back of his tongue before he is ready to swallow. In contrast, choking is dangerous. It closes off the windpipe so a child cannot breathe. Have your health care provider teach you first aid for choking. A child may also gag or even vomit when he is presented with unfamiliar food or textures. If you remain calm and don't pressure, your preschooler or school-age child can learn not to gag or vomit when he sees unfamiliar food.

- Always have a grown-up with your child when he eats. Don't leave older children in charge.

- Keep eating times pleasant, calm, and quiet. Have your child sit down when he eats.

- Adapt or gradually introduce foods that can plug up a child's windpipe: grapes, hot dog rounds, meat, nuts, raw vegetables or fruits, hard candy, jelly beans, caramels, gum drops. Spread peanut butter thinly. Remove fish bones.

- Don't get pushy with feeding. If you put pressure on your child to eat, he may gag or vomit to get you to back off.

Have family-friendly meals

You are no longer just feeding your child. You are feeding a *family* and including your child in *family meals.* While you need to be considerate of your child's immaturity and inexperience with eating, you mustn't limit menus to foods she readily accepts. She is growing up to eat the food you eat.

- **Have food you enjoy.** Put together what you enjoy and ordinarily eat and provide it for family mealtime. For you to have—and keep having—family meals, those meals need to be rewarding to plan, prepare, and eat.

- **Lighten up your definition.** A *family meal* is when you all sit down together, share the same food, and pay attention to each other. You do not need a table—a blanket on the floor will do—and the food does not have to be fancy. But the TV, computer, and phones have to be *off.*

- **Start by getting the meal habit.** Make meals your idea, based on food you usually eat. Don't just offer meals when somebody asks for food.

- **Remember whose meal it is.** It is *yours,* and you are inviting your child to join you. Sooner or later your child will eat almost everything you eat.

- **Make mealtimes pleasant.** Talk and enjoy each other. Don't scold or fight.

Prepare food you enjoy

- Eat what you are eating now. Just have it at regular meal- and snack-times.
- *Be considerate without catering* (Page 7).
- Round up the family to eat together.
- Let everyone decide what and how much to eat from what you provide for the meal.

After that, you might crave a little variety

- Add on foods, don't take them away.
- Include one or two foods that each person (generally) eats and can fill up on, such as bread.
- Pair familiar food with unfamiliar, favorite with not-so-favorite.
- Include fat when you cook and make it available at mealtime to make food taste good. Fat with food also keeps everyone from getting hungry right away.
- Let everyone—including you—pick and choose from what is in the meal and eat what tastes good.
- Don't try to please all the eaters with every food. Don't get pushy with feeding.

Are you ready to do some planning?

Keep in mind that planning is your *servant,* not your *master.* Get as organized about meal-planning as feels right to you. Remember, you have to keep doing it over the long pull. The goal is consistent *structure;* it is not putting you on a guilt trip!

- Know in the morning what you will have for dinner.
- Figure out meals a day or a few days ahead of time.
- Look for meal-planning strategies in *Secrets of Feeding a Healthy Family* and from other family cooks.
- Give yourself full marks when you provide a meal. If you sit down and enjoy your food together, you can cook from scratch, defrost it in the microwave, have food delivered, or eat at a fast-food restaurant.

Family meals and the overweight or obese child

You can *Have family-friendly meals* as described above even if your child has been characterized—medically or otherwise—as being overweight or obese. For the child of size, the same as for every other child, providing structured meals and structured, sit-down snacks is *the* critical intervention. Do not deprive in *any way,* and do an excellent job with feeding as described in this booklet.

What to expect when you feed your toddler

When he first started feeding himself, your child may have loved to eat and eaten almost everything. Now, his eating suddenly changes. He becomes skeptical about new food (even if you know he has eaten it before), eats less (because he grows more slowly), and says "no" to food (often at the same time as he eats it). Your toddler's erratic eating can trigger your trying to get him to eat. Don't do it! He will eat what the rest of the family eats, but it has to be *his* idea. The toddler learns by trial and error. So it wasn't all right yesterday to *beg* for cookies, but what about today? So peas tasted good yesterday, but what about today?

Relax. Despite outward appearances, as long as you do your jobs with feeding, over a week or two your toddler eats what he needs. He learns to eat new food, but you have to do time-lapse photography to detect it. He eats as much as he needs and shows it by growing well and being so active he wears you out! With your help and with a few skirmishes, he behaves at mealtime so you enjoy having him there.

The toddler's eating is quirky

Do your jobs with feeding, but don't try to modify his erratic, picky, fickle ways or persuade him he really *does* like something. Save your breath. Time alone will persuade him.

- **Erratic:** At times, he won't eat much—a few tastes, swallows, finger-fulls, or bites. Other times, he will eat more than you can imagine.
- **Picky:** He won't eat some of everything in the meal but only 1 or 2 foods.
- **Fickle:** What he eats one day, he ignores another.
- **Cautious:** If he has not seen it before (or *thinks* he has not), he probably will not eat it. But he sneaks up on it. He watches you eat it, looks at it, puts it in his mouth, and takes it out again.
- **Messy:** He drops food, smears it, gets it all over his face, and makes his place look like a disaster area.

Don't feed to quell the riot.

The toddler is at high risk for learning to eat for emotional reasons. Toddlers are active, unceasing in their demands, and prone to get upset. They are also learning to tell the difference between their feelings and their bodily sensations—whether, for instance, they are hungry, angry, or tired. You help your toddler to learn by doing your best not to feed him to calm things down or to make him feel better. Instead, stick to scheduled feedings, and address your toddler's feelings by giving attention, hugs or naps.

Avoid common toddler feeding mistakes

- **Limiting the menu to the food your toddler accepts or providing special food.**
  He is learning to eat the food *you* eat. Making special food for him puts pressure on him to eat and deprives him of learning.

- **Playing games to get him to eat.**
  He will play games right back. You will do all sorts of embarrassing things—and he still will not eat.

- **Asking him what he wants.**
  He does not know what he wants to eat until it is in front of him—and maybe not then.

- **Leaving out little dishes of food for him to grab when he walks by.**
  He needs to eat with the family.

- **Waiting to feed until he says he is hungry.**
  The toddler doesn't know he is hungry until he is *too* hungry. Then he falls apart.

- **Feeding on demand.**
  Unlike when he was a baby, your toddler needs structure in all things, including feeding.

Feeding stories: the toddler

Clinton was jerking us around

Clinton, age 2, drank (milk and Pediasure) or squeezed (food pouches or Go-Gurt) most of his food. Even though he ate pizza, waffles, pancakes, french fries, chips, and quesadillas, the therapist said his poor eating came from poor muscle function in his jaw. But Clinton's grandmother said that was ridiculous, that Clinton was perfectly capable of eating, and that we had to have meals and sit-down snacks and follow the division of responsibility. Well, here is one family that does what Grandma says, especially since she helps us figure out the cooking! We cut out the Pediasure, the squeeze food (except for an occasional snack), and therapist. Instead, we *Have family-friendly meals* (page 15) and sit-down snacks (page 26). Now Clinton is eating like the usual picky toddler, but he behaves well at mealtime, and we aren't driving ourselves crazy any more trying to find something he will eat.

Todd would rather eat than play

Todd, 2 1/2, always wanted second helpings or even thirds. The minute he came to the table he began begging for more, more, more. Even with big meals, between times he sneaked into the pantry to get food. At birthday parties he hung around the cake and didn't play with the other children! We could go on. Todd's weight was going up too fast, but for us that was beside the point. It was his *eating*. Turns out that we were restricting him, and he was afraid of going hungry! We were trying to get him to settle for one helping only at mealtime and not giving him snacks between times. We learned that children can be trusted to know how much to eat and started applying the division of responsibility. At first Todd ate a lot and even threw up a little after some meals. But now he eats erratically, like a regular toddler. At the last birthday party, Todd played with the other children!

Curtis refused to eat

Curtis, age 2 years, climbed eagerly into his high chair, apparently prepared to do his usual thorough job of eating. But this time, he sat back in his chair, crossed his arms, glared at me, and announced, "I won't eat." I don't know where he got the idea that his eating was *my* project! Since he was my third child, I had long since given up on any such possibility! It seemed I was supposed to say, "Oh, dear, you have to eat." But I could see that little gleam in his eye that meant this was an opening move in a contest. It scared me that he might not eat, because when he was hungry he got crabby, impulsive, and super hard to be around. But I knew I couldn't get him to eat, so I said, "that's all right, you don't have to eat. Just keep us company for a couple of minutes, then you can go." He looked absolutely crestfallen. It *seemed* like such a good game, and I just wasn't playing. So he sat a minute, and then he said, "I want some of that." He ate it and asked for something else, and something else until he ate his meal.

Brooke *loves* butter

Brooke, 18 months, *loves* butter and puts up a terrific fuss until we put it on her plate. She eats it by the handful. On Ellyn Satter's Facebook page, a lot of other parents said that their toddlers love butter too and they try not to give it to them. But that creates such a fuss that they give in and feel guilty. Ellyn Satter said that giving toddlers butter is okay. She explained that the fat content in their diets suddenly drops off when they are weaned from breastfeeding or formula to table food. Toddlers intuitively eat butter to make up for lost fat—and calories.

What to expect when you feed your preschooler

The preschooler remembers what you tell her, goes by the rules, uses language to learn, and knows she is her own person. She is more ready than before to eat unfamiliar food because she can talk about it, remember seeing it, is impressed by your eating it, and doesn't have to use it to fight toddler battles for control. But you are as important as ever, and so is the division of responsibility in feeding and *Family-friendly meals* (page 15). Your preschooler wants to please you, and you can shame her into cleaning her plate or eating her vegetables. Don't do it! It will make her feel bad about herself and bad about eating. Instead, sharpen your curiosity and hang on to your sense of humor.

Eating with a preschooler is full of surprises

- Preschoolers can follow directions and remember rules.
- Preschoolers eat with their silverware—and also their fingers—and use their fingers to load the silverware.
- Preschoolers might love a sandwich cut into triangles and not be interested when that same sandwich is cut into squares.
- Preschoolers wiggle and squirm and swing their legs and wave their arms and tell stories while they eat. They have too much energy to sit still.
- Preschoolers can't be fooled. If you do something to get them to eat vegetables, they conclude that vegetables are not so good.

Avoid common preschooler feeding mistakes

- **Limiting the menu to food she likes best:** She is learning to eat the food you eat.
- **Pushing her to eat or to taste:** She pushes herself. She wants to grow up, with eating and with all things.
- **Expecting her to eat food you don't enjoy:** If you enjoy green beans, she will learn to enjoy them too—some day. If you eat them but don't enjoy them, she won't eat or enjoy them.
- **Giving unwanted help:** Ask her if she wants help cutting her meat or pouring her milk. Support her in serving herself and passing food by using small-enough pitchers, serving dishes, and utensils.
- **Not letting her act her age:** The preschooler is full of playfulness and surprises. Don't expect her to sit quietly, think logically, or act like a little grown-up. But do expect her to be pleasant.
- **Letting her behave badly:** Don't let her make a mess on purpose, whine and cry, make a commotion so others can't eat, make negative remarks about the food... you get the idea.

Bethany ate from a short list

Four-year-old Bethany ate Oscar Mayer wieners, Skippy peanut butter (smooth), Dean's 2% milk, Wonder (white) bread, Kraft macaroni and cheese, Minute Maid pulp-free orange juice, Tony's crispy crust frozen cheese pizza. You get the idea. The foods were nutritious and just *fine*. The problem was being *stuck* on them. Bethany's parents had arrived at this short and ever-shrinking list after years of desperately seeking *something* she would eat. Meals were a hassle because Bethany often refused to eat even her favorite foods. As a tiny baby, Bethany had medical problems, and her parents were told, "feed her, I don't care how you do it." Recently, the doctor said that Bethany was all right medically, so the parents decided to change their ways with feeding. They read *Child of Mine*, and decided to follow a division of responsibility in feeding. Bethany quickly learned to behave nicely at meals, but she existed on bread, milk, and a few bites of her favorites that were on the menu. Her parents gave her a multivitamin mineral supplement and kept reminding themselves that she was fine. After months and *months*, Bethany ever-so-gradually started to eat other foods.

Feeding stories: the preschooler

Erica knew her limits

Erica, age four, had a passion for chocolate chip cookies, and I doled them out one at a time. Then she started sneaking them. I read Using "forbidden" food (page 27) and ran an experiment. I made chocolate chip cookies and put out a plate of them for snack. Erica ate three *big cookies* and asked for a fourth. I said to myself, "How much more can she eat?" She took one bite, put it on her plate, got down, and went off to play. Now that the newness has worn off, she eats one or two cookies, even when they are fresh, or none at all!

My friend's child is eating better

I recently had a friend and her five-year-old over for lunch. The difference in mealtime behavior between her five-year-old and my three (ages five, three, and eighteen months) was remarkable. My friend tried to get her daughter to eat, the girl cried and whined, and the meal was one long hassle! As she left, I handed my friend a copy of *Secrets of Feeding a Healthy Family*, and said as casually as I could, "This book has been such a blessing to our family; maybe you would enjoy it, too!" She called three weeks later telling me that since she has applied the division of responsibility, her daughter's eating behavior and even general moods and behavior have drastically improved. She said the key was having planned sit-down snacks (and no between-meal juice handouts) and not feeling responsible for getting food into her.

How I learned to stop worrying and love planned snacks

I always thought planned snacks were unnecessary and that kids should be able to get by on meals alone. I learned my lesson. Four-year-old Reece was constantly trying to keep up with his older brother. That created trouble at mealtime, because once his brother asked to be excused, Reece wanted to go, too. So I would say, "first you have to finish your meal." Reece would do it, but he would just *stuff* the food down and look totally miserable and jump down from the table with his cheeks still bulging. So one day, I said, "okay, you can go, but no more food until dinner time." He was happy to go, but around 4:00 he was *hungry* and *begging* for food. I stuck to what I had said, but believe me, that was a long two hours until dinner time! So I realized I had to start offering my boys a mid-afternoon snack. And it worked like a charm. No more insisting Reece finish a meal, no more 4:00 meltdown.

Quinlan keeps us guessing!

For breakfast, my five-year-old, Quinlan, ate three pancakes with butter and syrup, two sausages, a slice of bacon, a scrambled egg, and a glass of orange juice. The night before he had a mouthful of pizza and a carrot. For lunch, he had ¼ peanut butter sandwich, a few swallows of milk, and two slices of apple. Quinlan has always been big—he consistently grows at the 95th percentile for both height and weight—and is very active. How does he keep himself going? And the thing is, as a baby and young toddler, he ate so much of almost everything! Now this. Most of the time he seems to live on air, and once in a while he eats more that you can even imagine! It is challenging to follow the division of responsibility on both ends, but what else can we do?

What to expect when you feed your early school-age child

In his school-age years your child is enthusiastic and curious about food and takes initiative with eating, the same as with everything else. If you have followed the division of responsibility in feeding (and continue to follow it), he will have positive eating attitudes and behaviors:

- He assumes that there will be a family meal, that he will be at it, and that he will be pleasant while he is there.

- With less and less of your prompting, he will remember his snack and sit down to eat it.

- He is pretty good at talking and listening, but even then, he can't sit still.

- He uses his utensils more than he did earlier, but still uses his fingers a lot of the time.

- He is relaxed about unfamiliar food, tries it sometimes, and is polite about turning it down. The list of foods he eats is getting longer.

Encourage your early school-age child's skill development

- **Expect him to remember the structure of meals and snacks.** Snack is right after school, before playing.

- **After he takes responsibility for remembering, let him pick his own snacks from your list.** See *Have structured, sit-down snacks* (page 26). He still needs your help to get the snack and needs your company while he eats.

- **Let him help cook.** He can help wash fruits and vegetables, cut them up with a plastic knife, and measure ingredients. For more ideas, see *Secrets of Feeding a Healthy Family*.

- **Let him be a child.** His way of sitting on a chair is to wiggle, wave his arms, stretch, and rock back and forth. He uses his utensils more, but still uses his fingers as well.

- **Look for reasons for negative mealtime behavior.** Avoid pressure (page 23). Check yourself: Are you keeping after him about his eating? He will behave badly if you do.

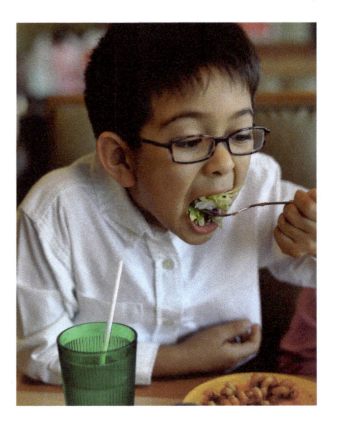

Feeding stories: the early school-age child

How I learned not to hassle Tucker about vegetables

Last night we went out for Chinese food, which my son Tucker *loves*. He was *so* excited. But before we got started eating, I said to him, "You know the rules—you have to eat your vegetables." I don't know why I hadn't noticed before, but this time I could just *see* how my saying that took the fun out of the meal for him. Well, I *do* know. I had just learned about the division of responsibility in feeding and how kids will learn to eat vegetables if their parents do and that I didn't have to be the heavy with vegetables any more. So I apologized. I said, "Tucker, I know you will eat vegetables when you are ready. For now, go ahead and eat what you enjoy." Tucker perked right up and ate a lot of different foods. He even ate some of the beef with broccoli stir-fry.

Cooper found his eating groove—for now

All of a sudden, Cooper, our six-year-old, has found his groove with eating. He seems to be growing fast and he eats a lot, compared with before. And he is trying new food: pasta with cream sauce (he's still not sure of tomato sauce), burritos, eggs Benedict (a passion!), Swiss steak. We have followed the division of responsibly through all of Cooper's challenging stages: Tricky to breastfeed, couldn't care less about semi-solids, ate enthusiastically once he could feed himself, didn't eat much again as a toddler and preschooler. So we will see what happens next! I am so glad we kept on doing our feeding jobs and trusting Cooper to do his eating jobs. I shudder to think what a feeding mess we would have created had we been trying to compensate for all his strange little eating behaviors! By the way, Cooper uses his silverware, but not always, and is so wiggly that he falls out of his chair!

Caroline eats a lot!

Since my six-year-old daughter, Caroline, has always been big and has an endless appetite, we tried to stop her from eating so much. Then I learned in *Your Child's Weight: Helping without Harming* that our restrictive feeding exaggerated her appetite and made her heavier. For almost a year, we have been following the division of responsibility, and her BMI-for-age percentile has gone from the 85th to about the 75th percentile. She still eats a lot (e.g., 4 to 5 bowls of cereal in the morning), but I have to trust that she knows what she is doing. On Facebook Ellyn Satter said to give her whole rather than skim milk so she has some fat with breakfast. Ellyn said research shows that children who drink whole milk are thinner, not fatter.

Clara's no-thank-you bite

Our four-year-old, Clara, is a super picky eater. It is hard on us, even though we have read Ellyn Satter's books and articles and believe whole-heartedly in the division of responsibility. Despite it all, we have occasionally tried the one-bite-rule with her when our anxiety got the better of us. Ugh. I don't think disaster is too strong a word, and of course I feel like a tyrant afterward, not to mention a division of responsibility failure. You can see the defiance and the anger in her whole body. She so reluctantly takes a miniscule bite of whatever we were pushing, makes a sour face, and then stops eating entirely at that meal and for a few meals afterward. It spoils the whole meal for everybody, and her older brother just hates it. So we learn our lesson still again. There is nothing we can do to get Clara to eat if she doesn't want to, and we must not try.

Your child's mealtime moves and yours

Even if he agrees to the rules ahead of time, your child will experiment to be sure the rules are *really* the rules. Your reaction can pull you into being controlling: into trying to do his part with the division of responsibility. At that point, your child is likely to become contrary and eat poorly. This table gives some ideas for how to stick to the division of responsibility in response to your child's experiments.

Your child's move	Your move
He says, "I am not hungry."	You say, "You do not have to eat; just sit with us for a while."
She is too worked up and busy to eat.	Spend a few minutes with her just before the meal reading a book or washing hands. Set a 5-minute timer.
He cannot take time to eat.	Arrange for him to be hungry by not letting him eat between times.
She is too hungry to wait for meals.	Have sit-down snacks between meals.
He is messy on purpose (he drops, throws, or smears food) for fun or to get a rise out of you.	Give him one warning, then have him leave the meal. Don't let him come back.
She does not want to stay at the meal until you finish eating.	Let her leave when she gets full. She will stay at the meal longer as she gets older and enjoys conversation.
He is naughty or otherwise disruptive at the meal.	Have him leave. He is full or he would eat—and behave!
She comes back right after the meal, begging for a food handout.	Don't give her food until snack-time. Ignore her tantrums.
He gets down, but wants your attention, to sit on your lap, to eat off your plate.	Pat him on the head and send him away. Teach him to play quietly while you eat.
She does not eat "enough" at mealtime.	Only she knows how much is enough. Don't let her eat or drink between times, except for water. Plan a snack for a set time between meals and stick to it.
He says, "Can I get the peanut butter? I can put peanut butter on my bread."	You say, "No, that is like making a separate meal. You do not have to eat anything if you do not want to, but you do have to settle for this meal."
She wants to make something different: "Why isn't that all right?"	"Because part of family meals is sharing the same food. You do not have to eat anything if you do not want to. . ."
"Why?" or "Why not?"	"Because those are the rules."

Troubleshooting with the division of responsibility

You are correctly applying the division of responsibility when you have pleasant, harmonious meal- and snack-times and your child wants to be there. She feels good about eating, behaves nicely at mealtime, and eats in a relaxed fashion. If you and she can do all that (and keep doing it), your child will consistently eat the amount she needs and gradually learn to eat the food you eat. If, on the other hand, meals continue to be a struggle and your child continues to be anxious or behave badly at mealtime, either structure is eroding or pressure is creeping in. Or both.

Set up and go by the rules with structure

Toddlers learn rules by repeated trial and error and consistent demonstration. Preschoolers and school-age children learn the same way and also by having the rules stated and explained. Your young dinner guests and their parents will be relieved when you explain your food rules:

- Food will be available at mealtime and snack-time. Other than that, the kitchen is closed.
- You do not have to eat anything you do not want to.
- You do have to say "yes, please," and "no, thank you."
- You will not say "yuck."
- There will always be bread, and you may eat as much of it as you want.
- When I make something new, I will also make something you generally enjoy.
- Sometimes I will make one person's favorite. Another time, someone else will get lucky.

Avoid pressure

Pressure is insidious. It is such a part of our relationship with food that it can easily sneak in to feeding. Pressure takes the harmony and pleasure out of family meals, and it always backfires. Trying to get a child to eat more than she wants makes her eat less. Trying to get her to eat less than she wants makes her eat more. Trying to get her to eat certain foods makes her avoid them. Trying to get her to be neat and tidy makes her messy. Putting up with negative behavior in hopes she will eat makes her behave badly but not eat.

- **Pressure can seem positive.** Encouraging, praising, reminding, bribing, rewarding, applauding, playing games, talking about nutrition, giving stickers, going on and on about how great the food is, making special food.

- **Pressure can be negative.** Restricting amounts or types of food, giving the *look*, asking "do you really want that?" encouraging, coaxing, punishing, shaming, criticizing, begging, withholding dessert, treats, or fun activities, physically forcing, threatening. Getting angry about your child's eating.

- **Pressure can seem like good parenting.** Encouraging or reminding her to eat, taste, smell or lick, making her eat her vegetables, warning her that she will be hungry, making special food, keeping after her to use her silverware or napkin, hiding vegetables in other foods, letting her eat whenever she wants to between meals.

- **Pressure can be hard to detect.** Ask yourself why you are doing something with feeding. Is it to get your child to eat more, less or different food than she does on her own? If so, it is pressure.

Making repairs

Been doing it all wrong so far? Feeding is a mess? Not to worry—we all make mistakes. Your child will change if you change—and stay changed. Review the material in this section. Agree with your partner on your plan, and be prepared to stick to it. Then, start working your way out:

- **Have a talk with your child.** "You know, I have been trying to get you to eat by (put your error here). From now on I will (how you will correct your feeding error here)."

- **Do it.** Be prepared for your child's eating behaviors to become extreme in all the ways you have been trying to control: eating more (or less), avoiding vegetables, eating vats of "forbidden" food whenever you make it available. (Add your key dread here.)

- **Hold firm with the division of responsibility.** Your child's dreaded eating behaviors will moderate.

- **Continue to hold firm.** If you let feeding relapse, your child's dreaded eating behaviors will come back in far less time than it took to get rid of them in the first place. And they will be harder to extinguish.

Food waste, young children, and the clean plate club

You may be trying to get your child to eat to avoid wasting food. Avoiding waste is a worthwhile goal, but consider other strategies—and consider normal child eating behavior. Food waste goes up when you feed children. Your child's hunger varies from day to day and meal to meal. As with everything else, he has a lot to learn. At first he may serve himself way more than he can eat. Encourage him to take small servings, show him how, and reassure him he can have more if he wants it. Don't make him eat it even if he only takes a little. He can learn to avoid wasting a *lot* of food, but don't teach him to clean his plate. It will teach him to ignore his hunger and fullness. Even adults can't always estimate ahead of time how hungry they are.

My five-year-old pressure-detector

It's easy to tell when things are getting off track with the division of responsibly in feeding my five-year-old. It has to do with pressure. She simply does not and has never responded well to any sort of pressure from us or anyone else as to what or how much to eat. Pressure immediately turns our mealtimes into a battleground, which I absolutely detest. I now love that she does not finish everything on her plate. To me, that says that she is attuned to her sense of satiety. And it is such a pleasure to hear her ask to try things of her own free will that she has refused for so long, and not because of our pressuring to do so. We don't always get it right, but we can depend on her to let us know when we've crossed the line from doing our jobs to trying to do hers!

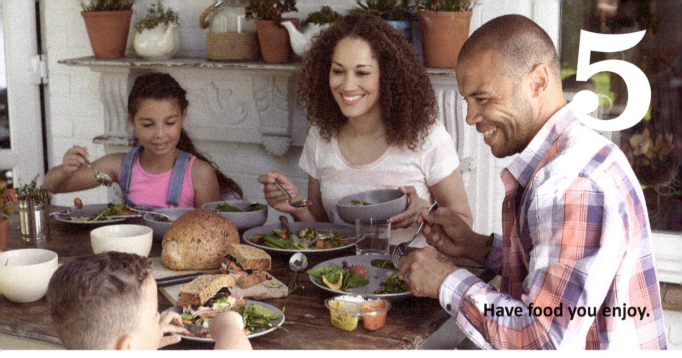

Have food you enjoy.

5. *What* to feed your family

As we emphasized in Chapter 4: "How to Feed Your Child," you are now feeding a *family a*nd including your child in *family meals*. You are no longer just feeding your child as you did when he was a baby. If you skipped ahead to this section, go back to chapter 4, and take time to master the principles of *feeding*. Nutrition falls into place when you have an excellent grasp of *how* to feed.

Meals are essential

For your child to eat well, you must have meals. *Have family-friendly meals* (page 15) reminds you that meals don't have to be difficult, drab, or unappealing.

- Have *family-friendly meals* (page 15). Establish the meal habit by eating what you eat now.
- Use snacks to support mealtime. *Sit-down snacks* (next page) between meals let children and grown-ups arrive at meals hungry and ready to eat.
- As you get tired of eating the same-old, same-old, add on a little variety.
- The next step, if you choose to take it, is to do some planning, perhaps even making use of the food groups.

Set realistic goals

Don't pin your feelings of success on your child's *eating*. The goal is *not* getting him to eat tonight's dinner. It is giving him positive attitudes about eating and practical behaviors around food that will last him for a *lifetime*. Use your commitment to good nutrition to guide you in your shopping and meal-planning. Don't let your commitment morph into putting pressure on your child to eat. You might be able to get him to eat his vegetables or drink his milk *today,* but not in the long run.

Consider using food groups

If you are to keep up the considerable day-in, day-out effort of providing family meals, those meals have to be realistic and rewarding for you to plan, prepare, serve, and eat. Basing meal-planning on food groups can put you on a guilt trip, or it can spark your creativity. You choose! For fast meals based on the food groups, see *Cooking in a hurry* (page 28).

- **Include all the food groups.** Meat or other protein; a couple of starchy foods; fruit or vegetable or both; butter, regular salad dressing, or gravy; and milk.
- **Always offer plenty of "bread" or some other starch that your family considers bread.** Because grains are easy to eat and good to fill up on, be particularly careful to include plenty of "bread" or whatever your family considers bread: sliced bread, tortillas, pita, naan, Asian pancakes or wraps, cornbread, biscuits, crackers, rice, or pasta. Although potatoes and corn are vegetables, they can go on this list.
- **Include high- and low-fat food in meals and snacks to satisfy both big and small appetites.** High fat would be butter, regular salad dressing, or gravy. Low fat would be fruits and vegetables (depending on how they are cooked) and bread.
- **Regularly offer high-calorie, low-nutrient foods such as sweets and chips.** See *Using "forbidden" food* (next page).

To learn more about food and nutrition without sending yourself on a guilt trip, see chapter 13, "Choosing food," in *Secrets of Feeding a Healthy Family*.

Have structured, sit-down snacks

Snacks are *definitely* not the same as food handouts or treats. Regularly scheduled, sit-down snacks are an essential part of feeding—and eating. See *Sit-down snacks solve feeding problems* (page 8). If your child complains about being hungry, tell him, "We just ate, but snack-time is coming soon."

- **Make the snack a little meal.** Offer two or three foods. Include protein, fat, and carbohydrate. See the table below for ideas.
- **Make it a sit-down snack.** Don't allow your child (or yourself) to eat on the run or eat along with other activities.
- **Let your child eat as much of the snack as he wants.** Trust your child to know how much he needs to eat, even when you include "forbidden" food (next page).
- **Manage amounts by managing timing.** Have a snack long enough after the *last* meal so your child is hungry and long enough before the *next* meal so he can be hungry again.

Plan a good-tasting and satisfying snack		
PROTEIN AND FAT *Choose from this list*	**CARBOHYDRATE** *Choose from this list*	**FAT** *Choose if you want*
2% or whole milk Hard-cooked eggs Cheese Luncheon meat Peanut butter Bean dip Hummus	Toast or another bread Breakfast cereal Crackers Cookies, cakes, muffins Popcorn Baked or fried chips Raw or canned fruit Raw vegetables Fruit or vegetable juice	Dip for raw vegetables Butter or cream cheese for toast or bread Fried snacks such as chips

What to provide for drinks

Serve *pasteurized* milk. *Never* serve unpasteurized milk of any kind no matter your child's age. Serve 100% fruit or vegetable juice. Canned, bottled, or powdered fruit drinks give fewer nutrients than fruit juice. Serve milk or juice only at mealtime or snack-time, not in between times. Don't let your child drink milk or juice whenever she wants it or carry around a container of anything except water.

Using "forbidden" food

Avoid setting up lists of "forbidden" food: high-fat, high-sugar, relatively low-nutrient foods such as sweets, chips, and sodas. Children who regularly get to have "forbidden" foods at family meals and sit-down snacks eat as much as they are hungry for and then stop. Children who are not allowed regular access to these foods eat a lot of them when they get the chance and are fatter than they might be otherwise. The trick is including sweets, chips, and sodas regularly enough so they don't get to be "forbidden," but not making them available in unlimited quantities, all the time.

Make wise use of "forbidden" foods

- **Include chips or fries at mealtimes.** How often you do this is up to you. Arrange to have enough so everyone can eat as much as they want. Unlike sweets, fatty foods do not compete with other mealtime foods.
- **Have sweets for dessert (if you like dessert), but limit everyone to one serving.** Put that one serving at each person's place. Let your child—or yourself—eat it before, during, or after the meal. Don't give seconds.
- **Offer unlimited sweets at occasional snack-times.** How often is up to you. Offer milk and a plate of cookies. Have your child sit down and let her eat as many cookies and drink as much milk as she wants. At first she will eat a lot, but later on she won't eat so many.
- **Have soda occasionally for snack-time or along with a particular meal.** If you drink soda, maintain a double standard. Tell your child it is a grown-up drink, which it is. After she develops a taste for soda (and she will), include soda with meals that taste good with it, such as pizza or tacos. Occasionally allow soda along with a snack that provides another source of protein, such as cheese or peanut butter and crackers.

Why is the sweets rule different for meals and snacks? Letting your child fill up on easy-to-eat dessert takes away his interest in eating more-difficult-to-eat mealtime foods such as vegetables. But at snack-time, there is no competition.

The sticky topic of Halloween candy

When your child comes home from trick-or-treating, let him lay out his booty, gloat over it, sort it and eat as much of it as he wants. Let him do the same the next day. Then have him put the candy away and relegate it to meal- and snack-time: a couple of small pieces at meals for dessert and as much as he wants for snack-time. Offer milk with the candy, and you have a chance at good nutrition. As soon as he can follow the rules (save sweets for meals or snacks), let him keep his stash.

Cooking in a hurry

Planning doesn't have to be complicated

Here are some nutritious, fast, appealing, complete meals that incorporate all the food groups:

- Spaghetti and meat sauce with grated cheese on top. (Or use frozen meatballs.) Bread and butter. Milk to drink.
- Cheeseburger on a bun (buy or make your own frozen hamburger patties) with tossed salad. Milk to drink.
- Baked lemon chicken (smear with butter, sprinkle on lemon pepper), scalloped potatoes from mix, canned corn, bread. Milk to drink.

Be ready to cook out of your food stash

These grab-and-dump meals are tasty, complete, and great for when you just *can't* cook. Remember to serve milk with the meal—it fills in nutritional gaps. You might have dessert—or you might not. It is up to you.

- Canned pinto beans or chili beans on rice with grated cheese, corn tortillas, and canned grapefruit slices.
- Tuna salad sandwiches. Hot tuna sandwiches on buns (foil-wrap tuna salad and cheese on a bun and bake 15 minutes at 325° F). Canned peaches for dessert.
- Hot dogs on buns, canned baked beans, canned fruit, and ice cream for dessert.
- Boxed bean dishes like red beans and rice (add butter or sausage for fat and flavor), bread, canned or fresh grapefruit sections or orange rounds.
- Macaroni and cheese (from a box), bread, and canned green beans. You can put tuna, hot dogs, sausage, or ham in the macaroni and cheese to increase the protein.
- Canned "hearty" soups with crackers, bread, and ice cream for dessert. Read the label to find soups that have at least 5-7 grams of protein per serving.
- Canned beef stew with refrigerator biscuits and canned fruit.
- Eggs, eggs, and more eggs: Scrambled eggs, boiled eggs, fried eggs, omelets. Toast, canned fruit or juice. The food police now say we may eat eggs.

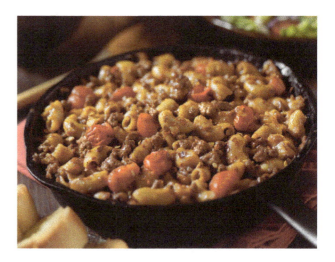

Consider easy casseroles

It is a myth that kids don't eat casseroles. They do, the same as they eat everything else: sometimes yes, sometimes no. But don't have a one-dish meal. Eaters need other foods—bread, fruit, raw vegetables—to choose from in case they can't eat the casserole. To get started with easy casseroles, consider *macaroni-tomato-hamburger casserole*, or *tuna-noodle casserole*. Look on the web for recipes. Don't worry about the salt in the canned soup. The soup—and the salt—get diluted by other ingredients.

Want more cooking advice?

"How to Cook" in *Secrets of Feeding a Healthy Family* helps you find doable ways to build your family meal habit. It gives lots of ideas and recipes for easy meals. It also addresses adapting foods for young children, and finding ways for kids to "help" in the kitchen.

Choosing food in restaurants

Most families eat out at least once a week. If you eat out only occasionally, eat what tastes good to you. Chances are, it will add up to a balanced meal. If you eat out often, still eat what tastes good to you! Also consider these suggestions:

- **You do not have to order food for your child from children's menus.** Menus for kids usually are limited to high-fat, easy-to-eat foods. To offer your child more variety, consider the appetizers or split a meal. You could also order an adult meal for your child and take any leftovers home.
- **Try for three different food groups.** This is pretty easy. A hamburger, a bun, and French fries give three food groups. So does pizza (crust, cheese, and topping). A salad, bread, and milk works, as does a taco (tortilla, meat, and vegetables).
- **Include fried food if you enjoy it.** Since many people don't fry at home, you may be eating out to get it! Food that is fried is still *food*. Following the three-food-group guideline will balance things out.
- **Limit sweets to one per meal.** A milkshake or soda is a sweet. To have dessert, have milk or water to drink. (For more about sweets, see *Using "forbidden" food* page 27.)
- **Keep dessert portions child-sized, just as you would at home.** That might mean splitting a dessert with someone else, or ordering a small sundae rather than a banana split.
- **Lay out cost limits ahead of time, then help your school-age child cope.** Order bread and let him fill up on that if he does not eat what he ordered.
- **Do problem-solving about waste.** Kids waste even more food than usual in restaurants. Don't insist your child eat it if he ordered it. Instead, ask him about it: "You ordered this food and didn't eat it. What do you think we should do about it?" Or you might say, "What do you think we should do about it next time?" One of his solutions may be to take it home, and eat it at another meal or snack.

Tips for grandparents who foot the restaurant bill

Decide how much you are willing to spend on your grandchild's meal. Don't worry about being a cheapskate. Assume that he won't eat it. Or maybe he will, but if you spend too much he won't eat enough to make you feel better. If he is old enough, tell him how much he can spend and help him figure out what he can order for that amount of money. Let him include dessert if he wants it. Ignore food waste. Do not feel obligated to get him something different if he doesn't eat what he ordered.

Fast food restaurants and the "overweight" child

Just so you know and can protect yourself from interference, child obesity guidelines say "limit eating out at restaurants—particularly fast-food restaurants." The writers of those guidelines assume that fast-food-eating causes child obesity. Not true. Almost all families depend on fast-food restaurants, and most children remain slim. Make wise use of restaurants—including fast-food restaurants—by *having family meals* and *maintaining structure*. There is a world of difference between whipping through the drive-through and throwing a bag of food into the back seat and going into the restaurant (or taking the food home), sitting down together, and having a family meal. Hamburger, fried chicken, pizza, taco, and other fast-food restaurants offer nutritious options for family meals, especially when you follow the guidelines for *Choosing food in restaurants* (above).

If you are vegetarian

Both adults and children do well on vegetarian diets that include milk, cheese, and eggs. Giving your child enough calories and iron is the hardest part. Here is how to put together a good meatless meal:

- **Protein:** Have dried beans, peas, lentils, nuts, seeds, nut butters, and soy-based meat substitutes. These foods give iron, as well. Eggs and cheese are both high in protein. Mash beans for your toddler. Be careful when giving your toddler whole or chopped nuts or seeds—he could choke.

- **Grains and starchy foods:** Have bread and another starch, such as potatoes, at every meal. Choose enriched or whole-grain breads, rice, and noodles to give iron. If you want whole wheat bread, the ingredient "whole wheat flour" should be listed first. Since young children can have trouble digesting too much fiber, and since cooked dry beans are high in fiber, serve whole grains no more than half the time.

- **Fruit or vegetable or both:** Canned, frozen, fresh, or juice are all okay. These give vitamins and minerals, including some iron. Include high vitamin C foods with meals; vitamin C helps your body use the iron in other food.

- **Milk:** Whole and 2% milk give children an important source of fat in meatless diets. Read the label to be sure that your soy milk beverage has as much protein, calcium, and vitamin D as milk. Since soy milk beverage is likely to be lower in fat, be sure to include other fatty foods with the meal.

- **Other fatty foods:** Use fat in cooking. Offer butter, margarine, salad dressing, avocado, vegetable dip, sauces, and/or gravy. Your child will eat more or less of the high-fat foods depending on how many calories he needs.

If you are following a *vegan* diet

If you are avoiding all animal products, be sure to work with a nutritionist. Cutting out *any* major food group makes it far more difficult to get all the nutrients you—and your child—need.

My boys needed more fat

We are vegetarian and my two boys, 2½ and 4, are allergic to cow's milk, so they drink soy milk. We are doing great with the division of responsibility in feeding. My boys take what they want, eat until they are satisfied, and ask to be excused from meals. But I had to give up on structured snacks because my boys wanted to eat all day long. The older one would cry and cry until I give him food. I asked Ellyn Satter on Facebook and she wondered if the vegetarian food is too low in fat to keep them satisfied between meal- and snack-time. She suggested making sure they are offered plenty of fat, and seeing if structure evolved from that. And it did! I am making sure to put butter and salad dressing on the table, cooking veggies in olive oil, and adding butter to steamed veggies. I am also adding more olive oil to hummus, offering guacamole with chips and crackers, and offering cream cheese or nut butter dips for fruit. And . . . they are staying full longer! They are no longer begging constantly for food and they are making it to snack times without melting down.

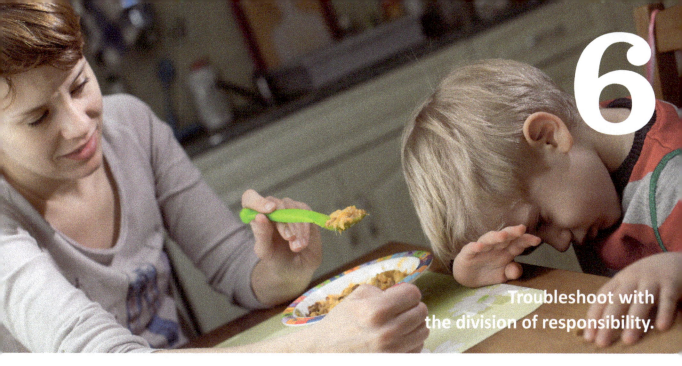

Troubleshoot with the division of responsibility.

6. Solve feeding problems

"My child is a picky eater."

Picky eating is normal, but *finicky* eating is a problem—with a history. You will recognize your child's history in many of the feeding stories.

What *picky* looks like

Your child behaves well at family meals, eats one or two foods, matter-of-factly ignores others, and eats a food one time but not another. She watches you eat, touches food, puts it in her mouth, and takes it out again. You might serve a food at as many as 15 or 20 meals or at *countless* meals before she eats it.

What *finicky* looks like

Your child behaves poorly at family meals. Any food not on her short list upsets her, and even when you make those short-list foods, she often will not eat. You get aggravated and try to get her to eat.

Finicky eaters can be born or made, or both

Some children are naturally sensitive to new tastes or textures—or to anything new, period—and may even be said to have "sensory issues." But even sensitive children learn to eat, provided they have chances to learn with no pressure to eat.

How to address finicky eating

When you do your jobs with feeding, sooner or later, on her own, your child will learn to eat new foods. *Stop* pressuring her to eat and *start* letting her be comfortable and feel successful at mealtime.

- **Have mealtime be pleasant.** Include her in conversation, but don't let anybody talk about food or her eating. Let her leave when she finishes; *have* her leave if she behaves badly.

- **Include one or two foods she generally eats.** Make enough for everyone. Let her eat as much of her familiar food that she wants, even if she only eats bread at every meal for *weeks*!

- **Make other food available and take "no" for an answer.** Teach her to say "yes, please" and "no, thank you."

- **Give her an out.** Tell her, "you can find something to eat, but you don't *have* to eat."

- **Maintain the structure of meals and snacks.** Don't let her have food or drinks between times.

Remember: Have family-friendly meals (page 15) and maintain a division of responsibility.

"My child will not eat at mealtime and then begs for food."

Don't attempt to solve the problem by trying to get your child to eat more at mealtime. He won't. Instead, support him in eating as well as he can at mealtime by being careful to follow the division of responsibility. Resign yourself to the fact that *The toddler's eating is quirky* (page 16). *Avoid common toddler feeding mistakes* (page 16). *Avoid common preschooler feeding mistakes* (page 18).

Don't say, "Why didn't you eat more? See what I told you—you didn't eat enough, and now you are hungry. Oh, all right, what do you want? But next time you have to eat!"

Instead, say, "The meal is over, but snack-time is coming soon. You can eat then." Then stick to what you say. He is learning that "no" means "no." He may pitch a fit. Ignore him. When he gets done yelling and kicking, the answer is still "no." After the storm, he will like you even better! After 2 or 3 days, he will learn to eat (in a child's typically quirky way) at meal- and snack-time.

"Isn't that a little harsh?" parents ask. "After all, he is so little and it is only one little cookie. What if I offered him whole-grain crackers instead? Why make such a big deal over it?"

Sorry, it *is* a big deal. *Your child depends on you to set the limit*. If you give in to his food-begging, the list of foods he eats will become shorter and shorter, and his behavior at meals will get worse and worse. Not only that, it scares him to get the upper hand with you.

Meals are about family and about sharing the same food at the same time. Everything else is just eating. Your child is entitled to learn that being included in family meals is special. It is special because he gets to be part of the family and because he gets to eat. *Be considerate without catering* (page 7), and teach him that to be there, he has to behave nicely and cope with the food you provide for the meal. Behave nicely yourself by not interfering with his eating jobs.

Set and follow a schedule of meals and snacks every 2 or 3 hours. At mealtime, always offer bread (or something like it). If all he eats is the bread, that is okay. If he eats a lot of bread, that is still okay. But don't get out the peanut butter, cheese, or the cereal. Those are different meals. Providing a separate meal tells your child, "I do not trust you to learn to eat the food I eat."

If the struggles go on, take another look at *Have family-friendly meals* (page 15) and *Troubleshooting with the division of responsibility* (page 23).

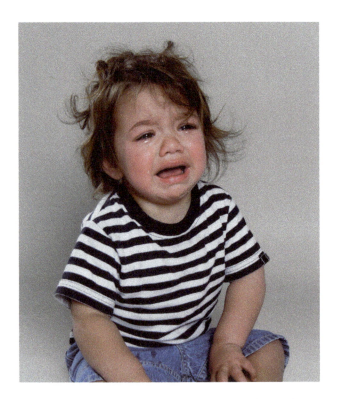

After the storm, he will like you even better!

"I worry that my child will get too fat."

To avoid or treat an overweight child, do an excellent job with feeding as described in this booklet. To make it work, you have to do all of it: no additions, subtractions, or edits. Feed your child like a normal child—which he is. Struggling to keep your child thin will make him fatter than is normal for him—and make everyone miserable.

Keep your nerve and do a great job with feeding

- **Feed in the best way.** Maintain the division of responsibility. *Have family-friendly meals* (page 15). *Have structured, sit-down snacks* (page 26). Even children who *love* to eat or eat a *lot* know how much they need to eat. They do, that is, when parents do their jobs with feeding.

- **Don't withhold food or try to push low-calorie food.** Don't sneaky-restrict or he will eat more and get fatter. (You know, *the look*, or *"what is your tummy telling you?"* or *"ahem. Do you really want that?"*)

- **Support but don't push activity.** *Follow the division of responsibility in activity* (page 5). Set limits on TV but not on reading, writing, artwork, or other quiet activities. See *Your Child's Weight* chapter 8, "Parent in the best way: Physical activity."

- **Recognize the signs of progress.** If you have been restricting, at first your child will eat more. But then he will relax around food and at mealtime, not be as food-preoccupied, ask for more food but not finish it, and begin to eat and enjoy unfamiliar foods.

- **Teach your child he has a good body.** Consider the word "fat" to be descriptive, not nasty. Help him find activities he enjoys and is good at. Appreciate his body, even if you have to address your inner weight bigot. See *Your Child's Weight* chapter 9, "Teach your child: Be all you can be."

Don't let anyone tell you your child is too fat. Studies show that, at every weight level, children gain too much weight when parents see them as being as being "overweight." Why? Parents of "too fat" children likely try to get them to eat less. Which backfires: Restricted children eat more and get heavier. Not only that, but "too-fat" children feel bad about their bodies and try to diet to lose weight. Which makes them heavier.

Trust your child to grow in the best way. Consistent growth at any percentile is normal growth. So is a gradual shift in growth over time. But abrupt shifts up or down could indicate a problem. Let your child grow in the way that is right for her. Read *Your Child's Weight* chapter 10, "Understand your child's growth."

You can't have it both ways. Trying to get your child to eat less and move more spoils feeding and destroys the effectiveness of the division of responsibility. For more about prevention and treatment of child overweight, read *Your Child's Weight: Helping without Harming*. Get help if you are stuck (page 38).

Owen's eating and weight scared me

My son Owen's well-child checks were all the same. "He needs to weigh less." "Don't let him eat so much." "*What* are you feeding him?" What can I say? I lied. Owen ate a *lot*. He hung around the kitchen while I cooked, ate a lot at mealtime and had to have snacks or he fell apart. It was hard. My sister is morbidly obese and I was so afraid Owen would have her problems. Looking back, I suspect food restriction made my sister so fat. In spite of my worries, I am happy to say that I did not restrict Owen but I did watch him carefully to make sure he didn't sneak and hoard food like my sister did. Now at age 23, Owen is a lean 6'3" tall, still has a big appetite, and gets crabby when he is hungry. It seems that what I worried about, his big appetite and the way he loved to eat, were just natural for him. Withstanding all that pressure to get Owen to eat and weigh less was hard on me, but I am so happy that I did the right thing!

"My child is too small or does not eat enough."

To address your child's slow growth, small size, and/or low food intake, keep your nerve and do a great job of feeding. Your child will eat and grow best when you follow the division of responsibility and concentrate on the *quality* of the feeding rather than the *quantity* she eats. *Have family-friendly meals* (page 15) and *Avoid pressure* (page 23).

- **Feed in the best way.** Don't try to get your child to eat certain foods or eat a certain amount. Don't praise your child for eating or scold her for not eating.

- *Be considerate without catering* (page 7). Pair familiar with unfamiliar food, include bread. Include fat, but don't load your menus up with fat.

- *Trust your child to grow in the best way* (page 4). Don't try to get her to be bigger than nature intended for her.

- **Recognize the signs of progress**. If you have been trying to get your child to eat more than she does voluntarily, at first she will eat less. But then she will relax around food, begin to enjoy mealtime, and behave better there. Over time, she will eat as much as she needs.

Be wary of labeling

Often children are labeled too small or "failure to thrive" (a scary term that means there is something wrong) when their growth is below the third or even the fifth percentile. Even without such labeling, parents worry when their child is unusual in any way. But don't let your worry make you put pressure on your child to eat. She will eat less and grow even more slowly. Trying to change your child's natural growth pattern will make you both miserable and is unlikely to succeed.

Crossing growth percentiles

Consistent growth at any percentile is normal growth. So is a gradual shift in growth over time. But abrupt shifts up or down could indicate a problem. To let your child grow in the way that is right for her, follow the division of responsibility. *Get help if you are stuck* (page 38), and *Consider a feeding relationship collaboration* (page 38). Read *Child of Mine* chapter 2, "Your child knows how to eat and grow."

Glory grew below the third percentile

Glory was always tiny, but she was healthy and strong. I followed the division of responsibility in feeding, she ate well, and my pediatrician supported me. But Glory had a bad cold at her 3-year-old checkup, and the doctor lost her nerve. "Glory's weight has dropped off and she doesn't look healthy," the doctor said. "I think you should get her to eat more." I pointed out that Glory was sick, she hadn't been eating, and she was a little dehydrated, so naturally her weight was down and she didn't look healthy. And even if there *was* a problem, I had learned that trying to get Glory to eat more made her eat less and took the joy out of feeding. Giving her extra high-fat food didn't work either, because she just ate less of it. I kept feeding in the best way and after a few days, Glory perked up and ate better. At the next checkup her weight was back on the third percentile. I knew I was doing the right thing, but it was *so* hard to go against my pediatrician's advice.

"My child will not eat vegetables (or fruits)—and I don't eat them much either!"

While vegetables and fruits are good for you, they are not worth fighting about. When you follow the division of responsibility in feeding, you and your child will survive and even be perfectly healthy without them. But it probably won't come to that. Prepare and eat vegetables because you enjoy them, even if you are the only one eating them. If you don't enjoy them, don't force your child or yourself to eat them. If you want your child to enjoy fruits and vegetables, you need to enjoy them yourself. If you simply can't be a vegetable-fruit-eater, be considerate. Do not make a big deal about not eating them. Let other family members enjoy them.

You and your child can learn to enjoy fruits and vegetables

You cannot fool a child. Studies show that parents who eat—and enjoy—vegetables have children who eat—and enjoy—vegetables. Parents who eat but *do not* enjoy vegetables have children who do not eat vegetables and do not enjoy them.

- **Apply feeding principles to vegetables.** Follow the division of responsibility, *Have family-friendly meals* (page 15) and *Avoid pressure* (page 23).
- **Sneak up on vegetables.** Your child looks but does not taste, tastes but does not swallow. You can look in the grocery store. Buy a little, prepare a little, taste a little, throw away a little. Take your time.
- **Try, try, try again.** Plan on 10 to 20 tries in as many meals—or in *dozens* of meals—to learn to eat a new food.
- **Don't get pushy.** Everybody learns better with an out. You can decide not to eat it, even if you bought it and cooked it.
- **Prepare vegetables and fruits the way you like them.** They can be raw, cooked until they are just tender, or cooked until they are really soft.
- **Prepare fruits and vegetables so they taste good.** Add sugar to fruits. Bake fruit pies or cobbler. Dress vegetables up with butter, cream, oil, bacon, fatback, white sauce, cheese sauce, herbs and spices, or brown sugar. Put vegetables in soups and stews.
- **Don't trick your child into eating vegetables.** It is all right to serve vegetables in soups, casseroles and other foods, but don't *hide* vegetables in the brownies, the macaroni and cheese, the pudding. Your child will catch on and not trust you.
- **Know that some vegetables are hard to enjoy**. People who are *super-tasters* say broccoli, cabbage, cauliflower, and some greens taste strong and even bitter. Tone them down with butter, salt, or sauces.

Your child will eat vegetables—someday

From the time Kjerstin was little, I prepared family meals, but she would not *touch* a vegetable. I knew other mothers were freaking out about vegetables, but my thinking was, "If she doesn't eat vegetables, I can't make her." I followed the division of responsibility with feeding, I prepared vegetables nicely and put them on the table, and ate and enjoyed them myself. I felt that was all I could do. The rest of the family enjoyed them, and none of us made a fuss about eating vegetables. Then, when Kjerstin was around 11 years old, she seemed to notice that she was missing out, and she started eating—and liking—vegetables. She did it all on her own. I think if we had forced or tricked her, she would never have done it.

"My child will not drink milk."

Children depend on milk for calcium, vitamin D, and protein. Children who drink soda or juice instead of milk are shorter, and they have smaller bones and more broken bones. You cannot make your child drink milk. But you can do a good job with feeding.

Model, but don't promote (or even encourage) milk-drinking

- **Drink milk yourself.** If you drink milk, your child will think, "That is what grown-ups drink." Even if she does not drink milk today, she will some day.

- **If you cannot drink milk, drink water.** Do not drink juice, soda, sweet tea, Kool-Aid, or other sweet drinks if you want your child to drink milk. At mealtime, let her have water as well as milk.

- **Don't get pushy.** Put a small glass of milk at your child's place, and let her drink it or not. Don't remind her to drink it (that is pressure). She knows it is there.

- **Don't go overboard with flavored milks.** Chocolate or strawberry milk are fine once in a while. But regularly flavoring milk to get it into your child is pressure, and pressure backfires.

- **Serve other food that contains calcium.** Cheese, yogurt, or fruit juice with added calcium give calcium. They may or may not give vitamin D.

- **Consider stomachaches or diarrhea.** If you are lactose intolerant, your 4- or 5-year-old child may become lactose intolerant as well.

- **You and your child still might be able to drink a little milk.** Try drinking a small glass of milk with meals. Try drinking 2% or whole milk instead of skim milk. Try a soy, rice, oat, or other milk-substitute beverage. Compare labels to see if the milk-substitute beverage has as much protein, calcium, and vitamin D as milk.

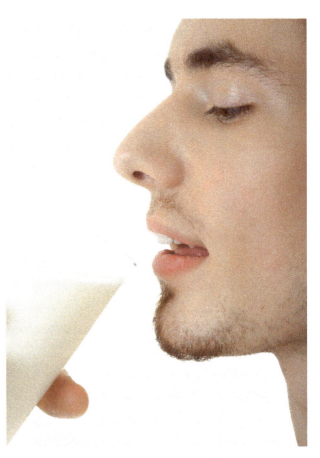

Your child will drink milk if you do.

My child will not drink milk

Following the division of responsibility was easy for me when it came to food, but then Jake stopped drinking milk! I worried about whether he was getting enough calcium for his bones and I confess I reminded and cajoled him a bit. Or a lot! I put Ovaltine in his milk, and sometimes that worked. But plenty of times he still would not drink it. I simply could not figure it out. He used to drink milk. Why did he stop? So I let go. I stopped bugging him about drinking his milk. I stopped flavoring the milk, and I started serving him both milk and water. Now things are much more pleasant at mealtime. When I recently asked him what he wanted to drink with dinner, he said: "Milk and water." He didn't drink the milk, but I took it as a good sign that he might start drinking it someday.

My child has special needs

The division of responsibility in feeding works for children with special needs, even children learning to eat after being tube-fed. When you follow the division of responsibility, even children with special needs push themselves along to learn to eat. But fragile children scare everyone, even experienced health professionals, and scared people pressure children to eat.

Respect your child's caution

Children who have had painful medical procedures that involved their mouths, or negative early experiences around eating, are naturally cautious about eating. Children who have been tube-fed early on have missed out on early eating experience, and eating is all new to them. But even cautious, inexperienced children *want* to eat—after all, *you e*at—and they want to grow up to be just like you!

Sensory issues are variants of normal eating behavior

Don't let your hands be tied by a Sensory Processing Disorder diagnosis. Everybody's got something about themselves that they have to learn to manage. Many children are temperamentally negative, shy, slow-to-warm up, so sensitive to tastes and textures they gag or even throw up, and react to scratchy clothing labels. Such children are *slow* to learn, but they *do* learn.

- **Establish a division of responsibility in feeding.** Feed your child as if she is a normal child—which she is. Be patient, but prepare to be surprised and impressed.

- **Work toward your child's feeling good about eating and behaving well at mealtime.** Don't try to get her to eat certain amounts or types of food. *See My child is a picky eater (*page 31).

- **Include meal- and snack-time foods that fit your child's ability to chew and swallow.** See Chapters 5 and 6 in the first feeding booklet in this series, *Feeding with Love and Good Sense: The first two years.*

- **Trust her to cope with her own sensory issues and anxiety.** Do your jobs, don't get pushy, teach her to be polite about gagging and vomiting (do it quietly, do it in the bathroom). With time, she will resolve these issues for herself.

- **Recognize the signs of progress.** Look for attitudes and behaviors such as enjoying mealtime, looking at the food, watching you eat, putting food on her plate, touching it, putting it in her mouth and taking it out again.

- **Understand how she learns.** She will not do, not do, not do, and then she will do.

Ava learned to eat at 18 months

Ava had esophageal atresia, a birth defect where her esophagus didn't go all the way from her mouth to her stomach. We fed her through a gastrostomy tube (a tube through the wall of her stomach) until her esophagus was repaired when she was 18 months old. Then it was time for her to learn to eat. On the dietitian's advice, we continued tube-feeding Ava, but we cut down a little on amounts to allow her to be hungry at meal- and snack-time. We got her up to the table with us and put little bits of soft food at her place. Once at each eating time, we said, "It's time for you to eat, Ava," and let it go at that. That was probably more for us than for her, because she watched us eat and seemed to know what was expected of her. After a couple of weeks, Ava picked up a piece of cheese and ate it. We were careful not to cheer, but what a grand day! After that, Ava ate more and quickly learned to bite off and chew. Before long, Ava was eating! To help us be brave about trusting her to eat, we kept the tube in for a few weeks, but before long, we had it removed.

Get help if you are stuck

Your child may have developed an established feeding problem. The problem has a history. Your child may have had temperamental, medical, and/or developmental issues that created negative feeding patterns. Such patterns attract negative advice that doesn't work or that makes matters worse.

You can tell when you are stuck

- Your child's growth veers upward or downward abruptly.
- You worry a *lot* about your child's eating or growth.
- You are making no progress toward having enjoyable, relaxed mealtimes.
- You and your child have prolonged or continuous struggles about his eating.

Consider an assessment

An assessment will restore your trust in your child to do his part with feeding. It is normal for your child to eat and grow normally. What got (or continues to get) in the way of his natural eating competence? To get answers, enlist the help of a professional who is expert in applying the division of responsibility. With your adviser, begin by doing an assessment that considers your child's medical history and growth pattern from birth, your past and present feeding relationship, your relationship as a whole, the structure of family meals and snacks, and your child's nutrition.

Consider a feeding relationship collaboration

Most feeding clinics use behavioral interventions that cross the lines of the division of responsibility and pressure children to eat. Instead, look for a professional who thoroughly understands the division of responsibility in feeding. It is best to have in-person help from a local professional who has been mentored and trained by the Ellyn Satter Institute (ESI). Because professionals who fully understand and properly apply the Satter Eating Competence Model and the Satter division of responsibility in feeding are currently a select group, ESI offers virtual coaching services. ESI faculty members and associates can connect with you by computer to help you find a successful and rewarding way to feed your child. You can find ESI coaching at *https://www.EllynSatterInstitute.org*. Your coach will help you to:

- Follow the division of responsibility.
- Feed in a developmentally appropriate fashion.
- At each stage, provide your child with opportunities to learn; then wait, wait, and wait some more. Your child will not do, not do, not do, and then do.
- Expect your child's eating behavior to become more extreme at first, and then it will moderate.
- Be entirely neutral, both in the way you present food and in the way you react to your child's eating and not eating. Be excruciatingly careful to *Avoid pressure* (page 23).
- Know the signs of progress. Your child will relax at mealtime, behave nicely, ask for food (and maybe not eat it), and forget about eating between times.
- Do *Troubleshooting with the division of responsibility* (page 23) when your child's eating relapses. Chances are, structure is eroding or pressure is creeping in.
- Be prepared for the long haul. Like other children, your child may be a teenager before some of his eating problems are resolved.

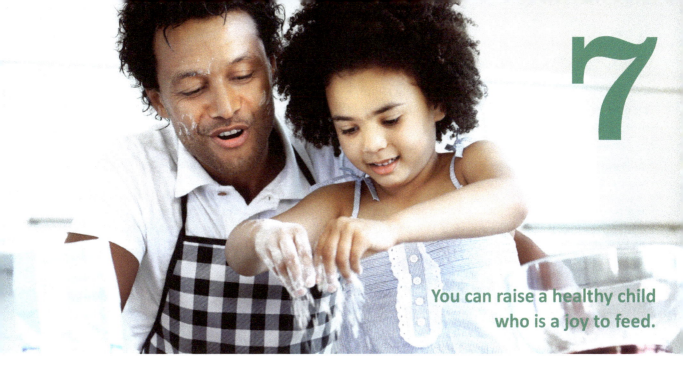

You can raise a healthy child who is a joy to feed.

7. What You Have Learned

Here is the bottom line: When you follow the division of responsibility in feeding, your child will be a competent eater.

It is all about control

You can control some things, you cannot control others. You can control what your child is offered to eat. You can control having pleasant mealtimes. You cannot control whether or not your child eats, how much he eats, and how he grows. Feeding is like parenting in all ways. You have to do your jobs, but then you have to let go.

Provide, don't deprive, and don't pressure

After you do your jobs, trust your child to manage his eating and grow up to be the size and shape that nature intended. Feel good about the child you *have*, not the one you *thought* you might have.

Check yourself. Are you doing a good job with feeding and parenting? Are you:

☐ Having regular, reliable, and enjoyable sit-down family meals? See *Meals are essential* (page 25) and *Have family-friendly meals* (page 15).

☐ Providing regular, sit-down snacks and not letting your child have food or drinks (except water) between times? See *Sitdown snacks solve feeding problems* (page 8) and *Have structured, sit-down snacks* (page 26).

☐ Being careful not to put pressure on your child with respect to his eating? See *Avoid pressure* (page 23).

☐ Regularly including "forbidden" foods at meals and snacks so your child doesn't overeat on them? See *Using "forbidden" food* (page 27).

☐ Trusting your child to decide whether and how much to eat from the foods you provide? See *Your child is a competent eater when . . .* (page 1).

☐ Trusting your child to be as active as is right for her? See *Follow the division of responsibility in activity* (page 5).

What Is Next?

Now you know most of what you need to know about feeding, and your child has become a competent eater. The principles in this booklet apply to feeding your child now and in all the rest of your years of parenting with feeding. You have established and maintained the division of responsibility in feeding. You have family meals. In the process of navigating your child's many changes in these early years, you have learned to trust your child to do his part with eating and growing. From now on, the task is for you to remain a good feeder, thereby letting your child remain a competent eater.

For more about feeding the toddler and preschooler, read *Child of Mine: Feeding with Love and Good Sense*. For more about feeding the school-age child and adolescent, read the next two booklets in the *Feeding with Love and Good Sense* series, *6 through 13 years* and *12 through 18 years*. See the back cover.

Your child can teach you about your own eating

- If you are anxious about your own eating, let your child show you what relaxed and joyful eating is all about. Keep your mouth shut and your fingers crossed and the look of surprise (or panic) off your face.

- Reassure yourself that you will be fed and that you can have food that you enjoy.

- Work your way through booklet five in this series, *Feeding Yourself with Love and Good Sense*, available at www.EllynSatterInstitute.org.

- Read more. See www.EllynSatterInstitute.org. Read Part 1, "How to Eat" in *Secrets of Feeding a Healthy Family*. Read the last booklet in this series, *Feeding Yourself with Love and Good Sense*.

To *raise* a competent eater, *be* a competent eater

Throughout his growing-up years, you teach your child to eat by the way you feed him and by the way you eat. When you sit down with him for meals and snacks and eat as much as you need, so does he. When you take an interest in unfamiliar food and gradually learn to eat it, he does too. When you respect your body and feed it positively and well, so does he. His taking good care of himself with food and feeling good about eating and his body are gifts from you that last a lifetime.

Reach out to others

Has this booklet been helpful to you? Would you like others to be helped to feel confident and relaxed about feeding? Here is what you can do:

- Tell a friend about it. Buy them a copy.

- Tell your health professional about it. Encourage them to purchase in bulk for their office by contacting support@ellynsatterinstitute.org.

- Tell your nutrition, health, or wellness teacher about it. Encourage them to purchase in bulk and use it as part of their curriculum.

- Talk about it on social media. Share your experience of becoming successful and joyful with feeding and confidently addressing your child's eating problems.

CPSIA information can be obtained
at www.ICGtesting.com
Printed in the USA
JSHW050752121222
34696JS00001B/4